Balancing Body and Mind

Integrative Yoga and Nutritional Practices

Table of Contents

Chapter 1. Introduction

In today's fast-paced, stress-laden world, finding balance and serenity can seem like a monumental task. That's where our Special Report comes in! 'Balancing Body and Mind: Integrative Yoga and Nutritional Practices' will be your comprehensive guide to igniting a harmonious, healthier lifestyle. Encompassing everything from accessible yoga sequences to science-backed nutritional advice, this report demystifies the path towards a fully integrated body and mind. Packed with expert insights, practical tips, and invigorating success stories, this engaging and down-to-earth report is like a sprightly companion cheering you on as you journey to wellness. Prepare to rediscover yourself, boost your vitality, and seize the day - all while nurturing a profound inner peace. So why wait? Dip your toes, or dive right into a wellspring of knowledge crafted just for you! Purchase this special report today, and let's embark on this life-transforming adventure together!

Chapter 2. Embracing the Concept of Integrative Health

The goal of integrative health is to synchronize body and mind - to holistically balance all aspects of one's life. Rather than focusing solely on physical wellness, this approach accounts for mental, emotional, and spiritual well-being. Here, we delve deep into the concept, its benefits, and precisely how you can adopt this approach into your own life.

2.1. Understanding Integrative Health

You may be asking: What exactly does integrative health entail? In essence, it is a philosophy that refuses to treat the body as a compartmentalized machine, instead regarding it as a complex interplay of parts and processes. By considering the whole person — physically, mentally, emotionally, and spiritually — integrative health seeks to understand and enhance human function and quality of life. It acknowledges that every part of us affects every other part, and thus, overall wellness cannot be achieved unless each aspect is cared for and balanced.

2.2. The Four Pillars of Integrative Health

When embarking on the integrative health journey, it's key to understand its four pillars: the physical, mental, emotional, and spiritual. Here's a glimpse:

1. **Physical**: This encompasses our physical body — everything you can touch, feel, and see. It's strengthened through exercise (like

yoga), a balanced diet, and adequate sleep.

2. **Mental**: This pillar refers to our thoughts and cognitive abilities. Keeping our brains in good health involves continuous learning, positive thinking, and regular mental exercises.

3. **Emotional**: Our feelings, attitudes, and perceptions fall under this bracket. Nurturing our emotional health can involve techniques like meditation, mindfulness, and appropriate expression of feelings.

4. **Spiritual**: Though often overlooked, our spiritual wellbeing is a fundamental aspect of integrative health. It can be cultivated through practices that help us seek and understand our core purpose and beliefs.

2.3. Integrative Health and the Mind-Body Connection

Typically, modern Western medicine has treated the mind and body as separate. Integrative health challenges this premise, highlighting the profound interconnection. A simple example is stress. When we're stressed, our bodies release certain hormones. Over time, chronic stress can lead to physical ailments like sleep issues and heart disease. On the flip side, physical ailments can impact our mental health, causing anxiety or depression.

Understanding this link, integrative health emphasizes a balanced approach to wellness. When nurturing your body through healthy food and exercise, you're inadvertently improving your mental health too. Similarly, tending to psychological wellbeing can impact physical health.

2.4. The Role of Nutrition in Integrative Health

When it comes to embodying integrative health, you can't overlook nutrition's vital role. Good nutrition does more than keep your body performing optimally, it also contributes to mental health. Consuming nutrient-rich foods can improve mood and wards off mental ailments.

Consider how the gut-brain axis operates, where the gut bacteria affect our emotions and mental health. A diet high in processed foods can disrupt this balance; conversely, a diet rich in fruits, vegetables, and whole grains can promote it.

2.5. The Role of Yoga in Integrative Health

Yoga is another cornerstone. Far from being just exercise, yoga is a mind-body practice that improves physical strength and flexibility while calming the mind and relieving stress. It can help build an intimate connection with the body, tuning us into its cues.

Postures (asanas), breathing exercises (pranayamas), and meditation are the three key yoga components. Asanas can boost physical health, pranayamas can aid emotional health by reducing stress, and meditation can support mental and spiritual health by fostering mindfulness and tranquility.

2.6. Your Route to Integrative Health

Embracing integrative health isn't about drastic life overhauls. It's about making consistent small changes that align with the four pillars, thus gradually creating a balanced lifestyle.

Begin with small steps: Eat a nutritious meal, try yoga, or start a daily meditation routine. Gradually, expand these practices until they become an integral part of your routine. Remember, the journey to integrative health isn't a race. It's about discovering and nurturing a lifestyle that works best for you.

Chapter 3. The Core Principles of Yoga: More Than Just Poses

Yoga, a practice with a 5000-year-old history, extends beyond the physical borders of movement and poses, known as 'asanas'. The essence of yoga lies in its core principles, which inspire a holistic understanding of the self — a harmonious blend of body, mind, and spirit.

3.1. Understanding Yoga: An Overview

To truly delve into the core principles of yoga, one must first gain a general understanding of the practice. Yoga is a physical, mental, and spiritual practice that originated in ancient India. The term is derived from the Sanskrit word 'Yuj', which means 'to join' or 'to unite'. Body, mind, and spirit unite in yoga to create an inimitable path leading to self-realization and mindfulness.

Although often used to enhance physical fitness, yoga is more than merely an exercise regime. It offers a comprehensive framework for human growth and development, fostering inner peace, calmness, and spiritual enlightenment.

3.2. The Eight Limbs of Yoga

According to Patanjali's Yoga Sutras, a revered text in the yogic tradition, yoga is divided into eight essential components - often referred to as the 'eight limbs of yoga'. These elements form the structural framework, guiding a person's journey through the practice. These are:

1. Yama
2. Niyama
3. Asana
4. Pranayama
5. Pratyahara
6. Dharana
7. Dhyana
8. Samadhi

Let's delve deeper into each of these principles and their relevance to modern life.

3.3. Yama: Moral and Ethical Guidelines

Yama is the moral, ethical, and societal guidelines for the practicing yogi. These are universal practices that, irrespective of nationality, culture, religion, or time, are pertinent. It is divided into five 'yamas', which are:

1. Ahimsa (non-violence)
2. Satya (truthfulness)
3. Asteya (non-stealing)
4. Brahmacharya (continence)
5. Aparigraha (non-covetousness)

These values align with many of the modern values deemed essential for peaceful existence.

3.4. Niyama: Self-discipline and Spiritual Observances

Niyama, the second limb, involves personal observances. They are divided into 'saucha' (purity), 'santosha' (contentment), 'tapas' (discipline or austerity), 'swadhyaya' (studying one's self and scriptures), and 'Ishwarapranidhan' (surrender to a higher power). These practices cultivate a deeper level of self-discipline, and aid in leading a focused and conscious life.

3.5. Asana: Posture

The third limb, 'asana', is perhaps the most well-known component of yoga, at least in the Western world. This revolves around the physical posture practice to care for and nurture the body. The positions are designed to build strength, flexibility, and balance, preparing the body and mind for meditation.

3.6. Pranayama: Breath Control

Pranayama is the regulation of the breath through specific breathing exercises. In Sanskrit, 'prana' means life force, and 'yama' means control; thus, pranayama isn't merely about controlling the breath but managing and channeling your life force.

3.7. Pratyahara: Sensory Withdrawal

Pratyahara, the fifth limb, is the practice of withdrawing from external stimuli and instead focusing inwards towards the self. It aids in developing a strong and resilient mind that can navigate life's hurdles with equanimity.

3.8. Dharana: Concentration

Dharana refers to the practice of concentration. The objective is to still the mind by focusing single-mindedly on a specific point (either internally or externally). It prepares the practitioner for more profound stages of concentration, notably dhyana (meditation).

3.9. Dhyana: Meditation

The seventh principle, Dhyana, moves beyond Dharana's single focus, and the mind becomes quiet. No single object of focus exists; instead, there's just a seamless flow of concentration.

3.10. Samadhi: Superconsciousness

As the ultimate goal of the eight limbs of yoga, Samadhi is a state where the self dissolves, and you become one with the universe. It represents a state of ecstasy and deep spiritual realization.

3.11. The Five Principles of Yoga According to Swami Sivananda

In addition to the eight limbs, it's worth taking note of Swami Sivananda's Five Principles of Yoga:

1. Proper Exercise (Asanas)

2. Proper Breathing (Pranayama)

3. Proper Relaxation (Savasana)

4. Proper Diet & Nutrition (Vegetarian diet)

5. Positive Thinking & Meditation (Dhyana)

These principles make the complex philosophy of yoga approachable and practical, unlocking a treasure trove of transformative potential.

3.12. Integrating Yoga Principles in Daily Life

Understanding the core principles of yoga is the key to harnessing the fulsome potential of this ancient practice. By integrating these principles into our daily lives, we can cultivate physical health, mental peace, and spiritual growth, thus, evolving into more balanced, wholesome beings.

To achieve this, it's crucial to embark on yoga not solely as an exercise routine, but as a lifestyle choice—a series of deliberate actions and thoughts that calm the mind, invigorate the body, and elevate the spirit.

Remember, yoga's transformative journey is slow but persistent. Be patient with yourself, respect your body, and navigate this glorious journey at your unique pace.

Chapter 4. Nutrition's Role in Balancing Body and Mind

Understanding the close relationship between what we consume and the impact it has on our mental and physical well-being is key for those seeking a balanced body and mind. Laying on food as medicine rather than just fuel opens the doors to better health, improved mood, and overall wellbeing.

4.1. Food and Mood

Perhaps one of the most direct ways we can see the link between nutrition and our body and mind is through the very tangible effects of certain foods on our mood. Biochemical changes induced by diet can influence neurotransmitters, the brain chemicals that regulate mood.

It's no secret that after a night of overindulging in heavy, greasy foods, we can often feel sluggish and foggy-headed the next day. On the flip side, consuming a well-balanced, nutrient-dense meal may leave us feeling energized and alert. This connection is not accidental, but rather a clear reflection of how our nutrition impacts our mood and energy levels.

One prime example of this connection is tryptophan, an essential amino acid that the body can't produce on its own and must obtain through food. Tryptophan plays a critical role in producing serotonin, a neurotransmitter known as the "feel-good hormone" due to its mood-enhancing effects. Foods rich in tryptophan include turkey, eggs, pineapple, nuts, and salmon.

4.2. Gut-Brain Axis

Groundbreaking research has revealed an intimate connection between our gut and brain. Known as the gut-brain axis, this bi-directional communication network links the emotional and cognitive centers of the brain with peripheral intestinal functions.

Our gut, often referred to as our "second brain," is home to trillions of microbes known collectively as the gut microbiota. Consuming a diet rich in varied fruits, vegetables, lean proteins, and whole grains can promote a healthy microbiome. This nutritional approach can profoundly influence mental health and play a critical role in preventing and treating mental disorders.

4.3. Macronutrients and Micronutrients

To understand food's role in balancing body and mind, it's essential to understand the role macronutrients and micronutrients play in our health.

Macronutrients include carbohydrates, protein, and fats. Each of these nutrients performs a specific role in Maintaining our physical and mental health. For instance, carbohydrates are the body's primary energy source, proteins are fundamental for cell growth and repair, and fats are essential for absorbing certain vitamins and providing insulation.

Micronutrients, though needed in smaller amounts, are equally important for mental and physical health. These include vitamins and minerals that assist in the production of enzymes, hormones, and other substances crucial for proper growth and development.

Understanding how to balance these nutrients in our diet is fundamental to achieving a balanced body and mind. For instance, essential fatty acids, like omega-3s from fatty fish or walnuts, are known to support brain health. Similarly, B-vitamins from whole grains, lean meats, and legumes play a crucial role in supporting mood and cognition.

4.4. Hydration

Water makes up about 60% of the body and plays an indispensable role in maintaining health, including mental functionality. Dehydration can negatively affect cognitive function, mood, energy levels, and overall brain health.

While the required amount of water can vary based on age, sex, weight, and activity level, a general recommendation is to aim for 8-10 glasses a day. Beverages like herbal teas or fruit-infused water could also contribute to daily fluid intake.

4.5. Mindful Eating

Not only what we eat but how we eat can influence our mental and physical balance. Mindful eating, which involves paying full attention to the experience of eating and drinking, can boost enjoyment of food, reduce overeating, aid digestion, and promote a sense of calm and control.

Try eating without the distraction of television, computers, or phones, savoring each bite, and taking note of colors, smells, flavors, and textures. Not only can this enhance appreciation for the food but it can also build a healthier, more mindful relationship with food.

In sum, the food we consume daily has both immediate and lasting effects on our physical health and mental wellbeing. By taking a mindful approach to nutrition, we can transform meals into an opportunity for nourishing the body, soothing the mind, and reclaiming balance in our lives.

Chapter 5. Digestive Health: A Cornerstone of Wellness

Understanding the importance of your digestive health cannot be overstated. As the primary interface between your body and the food you consume, maintaining a well-functioning digestive system is arguably the bedrock of total body wellness. From breaking down food for nutrient absorption to playing a significant role in immunity, the digestive system's far-reaching influences span across various aspects of our health.

5.1. The Digestive System: A Complex Network

The digestive system isn't just your stomach and intestines. It's an intricate network that involves various organs, each playing a crucial role. Here, we'll familiarize ourselves with these organs and their workings.

Your digestive journey begins at your mouth where the process of mechanical digestion starts from chewing. Saliva breaks down food chemically, preparing it for the journey down the esophagus. The mixture, known as bolus, then reaches the stomach where enzymes and stomach acid continue the process of chemical digestion.

The partially digested food, now a semi-liquid substance called chyme, moves into the small intestine. The majority of nutrient absorption happens in this 20-feet long organ. To aid this, the liver produces bile that emulsifies fat into small droplets, while the pancreas releases digestive enzymes that break down carbohydrates, proteins, and fats.

The large intestine, or your colon, handles the leftovers. It absorbs water and electrolytes from the remaining indigestible food matter and houses countless beneficial bacteria. These microbiota play an essential role in synthesizing some vitamins and short-chain fatty acids necessary for gut health. Eventually, the rectum and anus handle the expulsion of waste material.

5.2. The Gut Microbiome: A Hidden Universe

Dwelling within our gastrointestinal tract is a populous community of microorganisms—collectively known as the gut microbiome. This microscopic universe comprises bacteria, viruses, fungi, and other entities, with bacteria being the most extensively studied.

Recent research suggests that our gut microbiome impacts not just our digestive health but also our immune function, mental health, and metabolism. Disruptions to this community—termed as dysbiosis—can lead to problems like inflammatory bowel disease (IBD), obesity, and even mental health issues.

Maintaining gut microbial diversity is crucial. To do this, incorporate a range of foods high in fiber, fruits, vegetables, whole grains, fermented foods (yogurt, kimchi, sauerkraut), and possibly a prebiotic or probiotic.

5.3. Nutrition for Digestive Health

A balanced diet is key to nourishing our digestive system properly. What we eat directly influences our gut health, thereby affecting our overall well-being. Let's explore some foods that can boost our digestive health:

- Fiber: Dietary fibers are plant-based carbohydrates that resist digestion in the small intestine and reach the colon where they feed our beneficial gut bacteria. Foods rich in fiber include beans, legumes, berries, bananas, and whole grains.

- Healthy Fats: Essential for nutrient absorption and satiety, include moderate amounts of healthy fats—like avocados, olives, nuts, and seeds—in your diet.

- Lean Protein: Essential for cellular repair and the maintenance of body tissues, lean protein promotes gut health too. Sources include fish, poultry, beans, legumes, and nuts.

- Hydration: Water aids digestion and nutrient absorption. It softens the stool, preventing constipation.

- Probiotics: These beneficial microorganisms support our gut flora. Find them in fermented foods like yogurt, kefir, and sauerkraut.

Remember, dietary changes should be personalized to your needs. What works for one person may not work for another. Consider seeking advice from registered dietitians for a plan tailored to your needs.

5.4. Lifestyle Factors Impacting Digestive Health

Beyond nutrition, several other lifestyle questions can influence your digestive health. Stress can stimulate the gut, leading to discomfort and changes in gut motility. Regular physical activity is known to stimulate the muscles in your GI tract, promoting regular bowel movements. Further, insufficient sleep may disrupt your gut's regular activities.

Yoga, with its focus on mindfulness, can be an effective stress reducer and a tool for maintaining digestive health. Certain asanas (poses) work particularly well for promoting gut health, such as Pavanamuktasana (Wind-Relieving Pose) and Ardha-Matsyendrasana (Half Lord of the Fishes Pose).

By comprehensively understanding our digestive system and influencing factors, we can make more enlightened decisions that pave the way to wellness. So, let's celebrate this cornerstone of health by adopting practices, foods, and habits that have our digestive health at heart!

Chapter 6. Cultivating Serenity through Meditation and Mindfulness

Stress can often seem like an unavoidable part of modern life, but there are techniques available that can help re-establish harmony and tranquility in your world. Two of the most powerful techniques are meditation and mindfulness. By practicing these skills regularly, you'll create a calm inner space that you can retreat to whenever external pressures become overwhelming. Again, the goal is balance - between the demands of the world outside and the peace available within. Let's begin our exploration of these potent practices!

6.1. The Basics of Meditation

Meditation is an ancient practice with profound modern implications. While it has been part of various cultural traditions for thousands of years, recent scientific research has confirmed its numerous benefits for our physical and mental health.

At a basic level, meditation involves focusing your attention and eliminating the stream of thoughts that crowd your mind. This practice can significantly reduce stress and develop concentration. It can also encourage a positive outlook, self-discipline, healthy sleep patterns, and even increased pain tolerance.

Practicing meditation doesn't require special equipment or a particular location. You can meditate anywhere and anytime, though many people prefer a quiet, peaceful place where they can sit comfortably for a few minutes each day.

The most common form of meditation, known as mindfulness meditation, involves focusing on your breath while observing thoughts and feelings without judgment.

Begin your meditation practice by choosing a quiet, comfortable location. Sit in a relaxed position, either on a cushion with your legs crossed or on a chair with your feet flat. Close your eyes, and take a few deep breaths, paying attention to each inhalation and exhalation.

As you breathe, let go of active thinking. Start becoming a passive observer of your thoughts. Don't try to suppress or ignore them, simply acknowledge their existence without becoming attached or reactive. If your focus drifts, gently guide it back to your breath.

6.2. Understanding Mindfulness

Closely related to meditation is the practice of mindfulness. Mindfulness is about being fully present and engaged in the current moment. While meditation often takes place in a quiet, sequestered location for a set period, mindfulness can be practiced throughout your day, in any situation or activity.

There's a common misconception that mindfulness means emptying your mind completely, but it's actually about paying close attention to your thoughts, feelings, and sensations without judgment.

To practice mindfulness, start by choosing a routine activity, such as eating breakfast or walking to work. As you perform this task, turn your full attention to it. Notice how the food tastes, the texture of the bread, the sensation of your feet touching the ground. If your mind wanders, gently guide your attention back to the task at hand.

You can gradually expand your mindfulness practice to other parts of your day, like listening to music, washing dishes, or even engaging in conversations.

6.3. Benefits of Meditation and Mindfulness

Both meditation and mindfulness have a variety of mental and physical benefits. They can decrease anxiety, improve cognitive function, increase happiness, and improve personal relationships. They can also lower blood pressure, reduce chronic pain, and improve sleep.

By providing a state of relaxation, they can counteract the effects of stress on the human body, support your immune system, and promote overall well-being. They also offer a means of self-discovery, helping you better understand your own mind.

The benefits of these practices extend beyond individual health and can promote a more compassionate society. By increasing empathy and understanding, they can help reduce conflicts and improve relationships.

6.4. Frequently Asked Questions

6.5. Is It Normal To Fall Asleep During Meditation?

Many people, especially beginners, report falling asleep during meditation. While it's not the goal of the practice, it's a common occurrence and typically indicates that you're relaxed. However, with more practice, you'll likely be able to stay awake and focused.

6.6. How Long Should I Meditate Every Day?

For beginners, 5-10 minutes of meditation can be beneficial. As your attention span increases, you can gradually extend this time. Consistency is the key! Even a few minutes of daily meditation can have a profound impact on your mental well-being.

6.7. Can I Do It Wrong?

Unlike many activities, there is no "wrong" way to meditate. Every person's experience with meditation is unique. The most important thing is to maintain an open, non-judging awareness.

Ultimately, the practice of meditation and mindfulness is a journey, not a destination. These practices foster an awareness that will help illuminate your path, promoting a balanced, fully integrated body and mind. Embrace the experience, embrace the quiet, embrace the peace – this is your journey, your path to well-being.

Chapter 7. Demystifying Yoga Practices for Beginners

Yoga is a practice that has historical roots dating back thousands of years, offering a stream of benefits such as increased flexibility, strengthened muscles, improved posture, and enhanced mental well-being. Demystifying the act of approaching yoga as a beginner involves understanding the basics of yoga philosophy and beginning practices, providing a solid foundation from which to build your journey.

7.1. The Origin and Philosophy of Yoga

Originating from ancient India, yoga was traditionally a spiritual practice, aimed at the attainment of Moksha, or liberation from the cycle of birth and death. While it still retains its spiritual roots, yoga has evolved over several centuries into a comprehensive system involving physical postures (asanas), breath control (pranayama), and meditation (dhyana), each designed to foster unity of the body, mind, and spirit.

Across its many styles, yoga emphasizes the direct experience of one's self and the world around us, promoting mindfulness, compassion, and gratitude. Entering the world of yoga, you're not merely signing up for a different way to exercise, but embracing a holistic perspective towards optimal health and well-being.

7.2. Getting Started: Basic Understanding

Primarily, yoga consists of Asanas (poses), Pranayama (breathing exercises), and Dhyana (meditation). It is a balanced mix of these three components that constitutes a complete yoga practice.

Asanas are diverse and cater to all from beginners to seasoned practitioners. The key to doing any yoga pose is to focus on stability and comfort. It isn't about twisting the body into the complex forms one usually associates with yoga images. Instead, achieving balance and stability in simpler poses is the stepping stone to deeper practice.

Pranayama can be as basic as observing one's breath to more complex forms like Kapalabhati (Skull Polishing Breath) and Anulom Vilom (Alternate Nostril Breathing). These exercises control prana, or life force, harmonizing mind and body.

Dhyana or Meditation form the third pillar of a balanced practice. It demands tranquility and stillness of mind, teaching you to focus and enhancing mental discipline.

7.3. Establishing Your Personal Space

Choose a quiet, well-ventilated corner of your home, keeping it clean and free of clutter. Natural light and indoor plants can also make the space more inviting. Wearing comfortable, loose clothing is recommended for ease of movement.

Opt for a suitable yoga mat made of non-slip material. A thin mat can provide better stability for standing poses, while thick mats could be more comfortable for seated or lying down postures.

7.4. Essential Poses

Mastering a few basic poses builds confidence and foundation. Here, we walk you through some fundamental asanas:

- Tadasana (Mountain Pose): Standing tall with equal weight on both feet, arms by your side, and taking deep, steady breaths, this pose improves posture, balance, and calm.

- Adho Mukha Svanasana (Downward Dog): Supporting yourself on all fours, and then lifting your hips to form an inverted 'V', this pose strengthens and stretches the whole body.

- Balasana (Child's Pose): Kneeling on your mat, sitting back on your heels, and stretching your arms forward on the mat, this is a restful pose that is usually performed between more challenging poses.

- Savasana (Corpse Pose): Lying flat on your back, arms resting at your sides, and eyes closed, this pose is used for relaxation at the end of a yoga session.

7.5. Simple Pranayama Practice

Begin your pranayama journey by observing natural breath. Yoga stresses diaphragmatic, not chest breathing. Observing and slowing down your breath can reduce stress and be soothing. A safe practice for beginners is the 4-7-8 breathing technique: inhale for a count of four, hold for seven, and exhale for a count of eight.

7.6. Guided Classes vs Self Practice

Consider joining a beginner's yoga class to ensure correct technique and posture. Once you gain confidence, you can integrate self-practice into your routine. A mix of guided classes and self-practice can be ideal.

7.7. Consistency and Patience

Practice yoga regularly but don't rush. The benefits of yoga unfold over time and practice. It's not just about achieving a pose but about exploring your physical endurance and mental capacity.

Yoga is about a mindful journey of self-discovery, beyond merely a physical exercise regimen. As a novice, your journey has just begun - take it slow, stay consistent, and let yoga's wisdom guide you towards balance, strength, and serenity.

7.8. Misconceptions and Overcoming Challenges

When stepping into the world of yoga, it's easy to get overwhelmed. The idea that one needs to be flexible to practice yoga is a myth. Yoga helps increase flexibility over time. Moreover, yoga is for every body type; it is not limited to any particular age or physical condition.

If you meet obstacles along your yoga journey, return to the philosophy of yoga, it isn't about successfully executing a pose but about the process, the journey. In embracing yoga's principles of compassion, patience, and mindfulness, your path, regardless of its hurdles, becomes the destination.

Remember, yoga is more than just the poses; it's a life skill that contributes to overall wellness, teaching us resilience, patience, and the ability to stay balanced amidst life's ups and downs. Cultivate an open mind, embrace the journey, and remember - every yogi was once a beginner.

Chapter 8. Holistic Eating: Nourishing Foods for the Body and Mind

The relationship between body and mind has been long chewed upon by practitioners and philosophers alike. It's an integral part of yoga philosophy and the science of Ayurveda. But what role do our eating patterns play in this connection? More than you might suppose! This sub-chapter will embark on an exploratory journey deep into the realm of holistic eating – from identifying nutrient-dense foods that fuel the body to understanding how food choices influence the mind. We'll also feature a discussion about the scientific underpinning behind this approach.

8.1. Establishing The Food-Body-Mind Connection

Let's begin with a fundamental question - how does what we eat relate to how we feel, think, and act? According to modern science and ancient wisdom traditions, our dietary choices have a direct impact on our physical health, and they also influence our mental and emotional well-being.

On the physical level, the nutrition we get from our food acts as fuel for the body's operations. It provides the building blocks for growth, repair, and maintenance of our body's tissues, and it supplies the energy we need for everything we do. Our brain, being the organ that consumes a vast amount of energy, is particularly sensitive to the nutrients (or lack thereof) in our daily diet.

When it comes to the mind, recent research indicates a bidirectional relationship between the brain and the gut, often called the "gut-brain axis". This complex communication network links our cognitive and emotional centers with peripheral intestinal functions. The food we consume can affect this communication, potentially influencing emotions, mood, and overall mental health.

8.2. Understanding Nutrient-Dense Foods

Nutrient-dense foods are foods that contain a high amount of nutrients relative to their calorie content. These include fruits, vegetables, lean proteins, and whole grains. Consuming such foods provides the necessary vitamins, minerals, and other healthful substances with comparatively few calories.

Eating a diet rich in nutrient-dense foods can lead to a variety of health benefits. On a physical level, it can support proper growth and development, reduce the risk of chronic diseases, assist in maintaining a healthy weight, and provide energy for day-to-day tasks.

Mentally, nutrient-density can play a crucial role too. Food choices can help moderate our mood and energy levels, as well as our ability to deal with stress. For instance, complex carbohydrates release energy slowly and help maintain steady blood sugar levels, preventing mood swings and promoting mental health.

Incorporating a good mix of these foods into your day can fuel both your body and your brain, for holistic well-being.

8.3. Guiding Principles for Holistic Eating

Holistic eating is about more than just choosing healthy foods - it requires adopting an entirely new perspective towards food and eating. Here are some guiding principles:

1. Mindfulness: Paying attention to what, when, and how much you're eating can bring about a significant shift in your relationship with food.

2. Respect for Nature: Opt for organic, locally-sourced, and in-season produce as much as possible.

3. Variety and Balance: Ensure you're consuming a wide range of different foods for a balanced intake of essential nutrients.

4. Whole, Unprocessed Foods: Choose foods that are as close to their natural state as possible.

5. Intuitive Eating: Learn to tune into the body's hunger and fullness cues, eating when you're hungry and stopping when you're full.

8.4. Planning Your Holistic Diet

Now that we've established what holistic eating is, let's delve into how you can construct a wholesome diet. Inspirations can come from both Eastern and Western dietary sciences.

Eastern traditions such as Ayurveda offer personalized diet advice based on one's constitution and the balance of bio-elements. On the other hand, the Western approach recommends setting daily goals for different food groups, ensuring an adequate intake of macronutrients and micronutrients.

While both approaches have their merits, the key is to find out what resonates with you and aligns with your lifestyle and palette.

8.5. Embarking on Your Holistic Eating Journey

Taking the holistic approach to eating may seem overwhelming at first. But the truth is, every small step counts. Simplify the process by focusing on one change at a time - perhaps start by incorporating more whole foods into your diet, or by practicing mindful eating. Over time, these small changes can add up to create a big shift in your health and well-being, powering your journey towards an integrated body and mind.

Holistic eating isn't a short-term diet or a quick fix; it's a lifestyle. You may need to adapt and adjust as you go along, but the rewards you stand to gain in terms of increased vitality and profoundly improved quality of life are priceless. Let this be your guide and inspiration as you embark on this transformative nutritional journey.

In the upcoming sub-chapters, we delve into the practical elements of holistic eating - breaking down the science behind nutrient timing, understanding superfoods, ethical and sustainable eating, and much more. Stay tuned and journey with us on this adventure towards true vitality and wellness!

Chapter 9. Boosting Internal Energy Through Pranayama Techniques

Pranayama, derived from Sanskrit words 'Prana' (life force) and 'Ayama' (control), is an ancient yoga practice focusing on breath control. Whether you're new to pranayama or looking for ways to enhance your existing practice, let's dive into this comprehensive exploration of techniques that can help boost your internal energy.

9.1. Understanding Pranayama

Breath is the bridge connecting the body and mind. By mastering the breath, one can increase life force, regulate bodily processes, and enhance mental well-being. Pranayama utilises a variety of breathing techniques, each offering unique benefits that effectively contribute to a more energized and balanced state of being.

It's crucial to become attuned with your body and discern what it requires. Each pranayama might have varying impacts at different times and circumstances. Be open to experiment, keeping in mind that what works best may differ from day to day.

9.2. The Power of Breathing

Listed below are some of the profound benefits associated with the regular practice of pranayama:

- Boosts energy levels

- Enhances mental clarity and focus

- Regulates the nervous system

- Combats stress and anxiety

- Boosts immunity

- Promotes better sleep

Let's delve into specific pranayama techniques to rejuvenate the body and mind.

9.3. Pranayama Techniques for Energy Boosting

Before you begin, sit comfortably on a yoga mat with your spine erect. You may sit cross-legged, in Vajrasana, or on a chair if you prefer. Keep the body relaxed, close your eyes and bring your awareness to your breath.

9.3.1. 1. Bhastrika Pranayama (Bellows Breath)

Bhastrika is a revitalizing breathing technique, involving active inhalation and exhalation. As a potent energy booster, Bhastrika is akin to fanning a flame within your body.

How to Practice: * Inhale deeply through your nostrils, filling your lungs to their maximum capacity. * Exhale forcefully, but not uncomfortably so, through your nostrils, emptying your lungs completely. * Continue this for 30 seconds to 1 minute. * With regular practice, you may gradually increase the duration.

In addition to boosting energy, Bhastrika can also improve circulation, relax the mind, and increase body heat, making it a great practice for colder days.

9.3.2. 2. Kapalabhati Pranayama (Skull Shining Breath)

Kapalabhati is a dynamic cleansing technique that purifies the frontal region of the brain and stimulates the nervous system. It's an incredible technique for an energy surge.

How to Practice: * Sit comfortably and inhale passively. * Contract the abdominal muscles to exhale forcefully through the nostrils. * Let the inhalation come naturally while focusing on the forceful exhalation. * Aim to complete around 30 rounds per minute, gradually increasing with practice.

Beyond energy boosting, Kapalabhati may benefit digestion, improve lung capacity, and increase metabolic rate.

9.3.3. 3. Nadi Shodhana Pranayama (Alternate Nostril Breathing)

While Nadi Shodhana might feel calming initially, it effectively cultivates clarity and invigorates the body/mind, bringing energy into balance.

How to Practice: * Using your right hand, place the thumb on the right nostril, the ring finger and little finger on the left nostril. The index and middle fingers can be folded into your palm. * Close your right nostril and inhale through the left nostril. * Close the left nostril, open the right nostril, and exhale. * Keeping the left nostril closed, inhale through your right nostril. * Close the right nostril, open the left, and exhale. * This forms one round. Begin with 5 rounds and progressively increase with practice.

Nadi Shodhana assists with cleansing and balancing the energy channels, promoting mental tranquillity and alertness.

9.4. When to Practice Pranayama

Pranayama can be practiced at any time, but early morning and around sunset are considered ideal as the body and mind are in a naturally tranquil state. However, what's most important is to find and maintain consistent practice, integrating these breathing exercises into your daily routine.

9.5. Tips for Successful Pranayama Practice

- Patience is key. Don't rush, take slow, deep breaths.

- Start slow. Increase the duration as you gain comfort.

- A quiet and clutter-free space enhances focus.

- An empty stomach makes breathing exercises comfortable.

- Be consistent for significant results.

Incorporating pranayama into your daily routine can significantly shapeshift your energy states. As you work diligently through these exercises, remember to listen to your body and mind, adapting the practice to what feels best for you. Embarking on the path of pranayama can profoundly impact your health, keeping you energized, focused, and balanced both physically and mentally.

Chapter 10. The Influence of Yoga & Nutrition on Emotional Well-being

Life circumstances fluctuate, affecting our mood and emotions every day. The ebb and flow can sometimes jettison us on a rollercoaster ride, brimming with highs and lows, and lacking equilibrium. Fortunately, tools like yoga and nutrition can make navigating these emotional landscapes smoother, leading us towards a stabilised and harmonious state of well-being.

10.1. Yoga: An Integrative Tool for Emotional Balance

In our constantly connected world, finding a personal sanctuary can seem elusive. Yoga, a centuries-old mind-body practice, can bring that sanctuary within reach, aiding us in fostering emotional balance. Rooted in ancient Indian philosophy, yoga involves a combination of postures (asanas), controlled breathing exercises (pranayama), and meditation. These practices aim to seamlessly unite your physical, mental, and emotional states, enriching overall well-being.

Postures, or asanas, are physical yoga positions that improve flexibility, strength, and bodily balance. Their effects, however, extend further than just physical enhancement. When you hold an asana, you consciously take your body into an unfamiliar position, which requires concentration, patience, and self-compassion. By translating this practice to daily life scenarios, we learn to respond to stressors with grace rather than react impulsively.

Similarly, pranayama, managing life energy via controlled breathing, features at the heart of yoga practice. It aids in quietening the mind, cooling the emotions, and curbing stress responses. Further, breathing practices are linked positively with mental health outcomes, reducing symptoms of stress, anxiety, and depression.

Meditation, another cornerstone of yoga, is a process of calming the mind and achieving clarity of thought. A regular practice decreases mental clutter, allowing us to better connect with our emotions without judgment. Through meditation, we learn to sit with our feelings, fostering mindfulness and emotional regulation in the process.

10.2. The Gut-Brain Connection: Nutritional Impact on Emotion

In addition to yoga, our diet is another significant aspect of emotional well-being. Nutrition affects our emotions via the gut-brain axis, a communication highway linking your digestive tract and your brain. This fascinating connection implies that our dietary choices impact not only our physical health but also our emotional state.

For example, gut bacteria play a vital role in producing serotonin, a neurotransmitter associated with feelings of happiness and well-being. A diet rich in fermented foods, fiber, and omega-3 fatty acids helps cultivate a diverse microbial population, promoting serotonin production.

Additionally, foods rich in B vitamins, such as whole grains, lean meats, or leafy greens, aid in regulating mood and warding off symptoms of depression. Similarly, the amino acid tryptophan, present in foods like poultry, eggs, and bananas, plays a significant role in the production of serotonin.

Omega-3 fatty acids, found in fatty fish, flaxseeds, and walnuts, have been linked to maintaining low levels of depression due to their considerable contribution to brain health. Ultimately, food isn't just fuel; it's a powerful mood enhancer. Emotional stability thrives under a balanced diet.

10.3. Bringing It All Together: The Symbiotic Relationship of Yoga & Nutrition

Yoga and nutrition don't exist in separate silos; they each contribute to a holistic model of emotional well-being. The mindful aspect of yoga encourages thoughtful engagement with our nutritional habits, helping us forge a healthier relationship with food.

Conversely, our dietary choices impact our yoga practice. For instance, a body nourished with balanced nutrition can perform yoga asanas with better strength, flexibility, and endurance. Further, the enhanced mind-body connection fostered by consistent yoga practice helps identify any unpleasant body reactions to particular foods, encouraging a more individualised and health-driven approach to diet.

In conclusion, nurturing our emotional well-being is a journey, not a destination. By incorporating yoga and mindful nutrition into our daily lives, we prime ourselves to navigate life's ups and downs with equanimity and resilience. These two interconnected practices create a ripple effect impacting our emotional health positively and leading us on a path to harmonious, integrated well-being. The journey may be challenging, but the outcome is profoundly rewarding.

Chapter 11. Creating a Sustainable Integrative Health Routine

Creating a sustainable integrative health routine is about more than just matching your yoga practice with a well-balanced diet – it's about adopting practices that become second nature, setting objectives that can be accomplished, and aiming for personal growth, all while upholding respect for individual circumstances and limits.

11.1. Your Personal Objective: Start Small and Build Up

Your fitness and health journey starts with defining your personal objectives. These can be as simple as wanting to feel more energetic, reduce stress, lose weight, or integrate more mindful practices into your life.

Once your core objectives are set, remember not to rush into things. Change never happens overnight. Don't set out to do an hour's worth of yoga and consume a completely raw, organic diet from day one.

Start with small steps: maybe 10 minutes of gentle yoga exercises or meditation in a day, and one meal adjusted to your new dietary guidelines. These small changes will gradually pattern into daily habits, making the transition smoother and more manageable.

11.2. Intuitive Eating: A Primer

Don't think of this as a diet, but more as an understanding of your body's needs. Our bodies often know what they need – the trick is to understand the signals.

Avoid labeling foods as 'good' or 'bad'. Instead, use your knowledge of nutrition to make informed decisions that support your overall health.

Keep a food diary that logs what you eat and how you feel afterwards. This simple tool can help you to recognize patterns and understand how different foods affect your energy and mood.

11.3. Incorporative Yoga Session

Start by incorporating short, 15-minute yoga sessions into your routine. Choose a time of day when you can consistently set aside this time – it could be the first thing in the morning or as a wind-down routine before going to bed.

The beauty of yoga is that it caters to all levels of physical fitness. You can start with gentle, restorative poses which primarily focus on calming your mind and balancing your body. Pranayamas, or breath-control exercises, can be extremely beneficial to manage anxiety and stress, promoting a sense of peace and balance.

11.4. Goals and Progress Tracking

To maintain momentum and commitment, set landmarks for your progress. They can be as simple as "meditate for 10 minutes daily" or "master the crow pose in 4 weeks". Use a journal or an app to track these goals. You'll receive a boost of gratification every time you achieve one, thus strengthening your resolve.

11.5. Listen to Your Body and Be Flexible

Your routine might not look the same every week. Some days you might want to push for an intense yoga session, on other days, your body might ask for restorative and relaxing postures.

Remember: absences don't represent failure. As long as you sustain overall consistency, occasional rest periods can be just as important for progress.

11.6. Remember, It's a Journey

This might seem like a lot to take in, but remember that it's about making changes one day at a time. As you become more proficient with your basic routine, you can gradually integrate more advanced yoga poses or dietary practices.

These expanded elements will come naturally with time. Be patient with yourself, learn to enjoy the process, and trust that the benefits of a balanced body and mind are well worth the effort.

Remember, a journey of a thousand miles begins with a single step. Start your journey towards integrative health today.

11.7. Seek Expert Guidance

Never hesitate to seek professional advice if you find yourself overwhelmed. Nutritionists can provide personalized guidance suited for your dietary needs. Similarly, professional yoga trainers can offer a personalized sequence that targets your objectives, adjusting it as necessary.

In conclusion, creating a sustainable integrative health routine is a rewarding journey of patient discovery, one that provides the tools to build a healthier body and a more peaceful mind. You're not just adopting new habits but rewriting your relationship with health and wellness. So embark on this journey with a positive mindset, patient dedication, and the knowledge that each step, however small, is integral to your personal growth.